# A

# Narrative literature review

# On

# GESTATIONAL DIABETES MELLITUS

**By:**

**Dr. Amitosh Kumar**

**M.D. Physician**

# ACKNOWLEDGEMENT

I would like to express my sincere gratitude and appreciation to Dr. Sayantan Chakraborty for his invaluable guidance and support throughout the process of writing this narrative literature review. His expertise, patience and insightful feedback have been instrumental in shaping and refining my work. I am truly grateful for his continuous encouragement and the time he dedicated to reviewing my progress, providing valuable suggestions and offering guidance to overcome challenges.

Lastly, I am grateful to my family and friends for their unwavering support, encouragement and understanding throughout this academic endeavor.

Thank you all for your contributions, guidance and encouragement. I am truly honored and privileged to have had the opportunity to work under the guidance of Dr. Sayantan Chakraborty.

# TABLE OF CONTENTS

**Abstract**

Gestational Diabetes Mellitus (GDM) is a prevalent condition characterized by elevated blood sugar levels during pregnancy. It poses significant risks to both the mother and the fetus and increases the long-term risk of developing type 2 diabetes. This narrative review aims to provide a comprehensive overview of GDM, encompassing its epidemiology, risk factors, pathophysiology, diagnostic criteria, complications, management strategies, and prevention approaches. Furthermore, the review highlights recent advancements in the field and identifies key areas that require further research to enhance our understanding and management of GDM.

Gestational Diabetes Mellitus affects approximately 7% of pregnancies worldwide, with significant regional and ethnic variations. The risk factors for developing GDM include advanced maternal age, obesity, a family history of diabetes, previous history of GDM, polycystic ovary syndrome, and certain ethnic backgrounds. The pathophysiology of GDM involves insulin resistance due to hormonal changes during pregnancy, leading to impaired glucose regulation.

Diagnosis of GDM is typically based on the oral glucose tolerance test (OGTT) and requires the presence of hyperglycemia with onset or first recognition during pregnancy. The complications associated with GDM include an increased risk of preeclampsia, cesarean delivery, macrosomia (large birth weight), neonatal hypoglycemia, and subsequent development of type 2 diabetes in both the mother and the child.

Management of GDM involves lifestyle modifications, including a balanced diet, regular physical activity, and weight management. In some cases, insulin or other glucose-lowering medications may be required. Regular monitoring of blood glucose levels and prenatal care are crucial for optimizing outcomes. Additionally, breastfeeding, postpartum glucose screening, and long-term follow-up play essential roles in preventing or delaying the onset of type 2 diabetes in women with a history of GDM.

Recent advancements in the field of GDM research include studies on the role of genetics, gut microbiota, and novel biomarkers in predicting and managing GDM. Additionally, technological innovations such as continuous glucose monitoring systems and telemedicine have shown promise in improving GDM management and patient outcomes.

Despite the progress made, there are still gaps in our understanding of GDM. Further research is needed to elucidate the mechanisms underlying GDM development, identify effective prevention strategies, explore the impact of GDM on offspring's long-term health, and evaluate the cost-effectiveness of various management approaches. Addressing these gaps will aid in developing targeted interventions and improving the health outcomes of women with GDM and their children.

In conclusion, this narrative review provides a comprehensive overview of GDM, highlighting its epidemiology, risk factors, pathophysiology, diagnostic criteria, complications, management strategies, and prevention approaches. By understanding the complexities of GDM and addressing the research gaps, healthcare professionals can enhance their ability to prevent, diagnose, and manage this condition effectively, ultimately improving the health outcomes for women and their children.

## Introduction

Gestational Diabetes Mellitus (GDM) is a condition characterized by elevated blood sugar levels during pregnancy. It is a significant public health concern, affecting approximately 7% of pregnancies worldwide. The prevalence of GDM varies across different populations and is influenced by various factors such as age, ethnicity, and obesity rates.

GDM poses risks to both the mother and the fetus. Pregnant women with GDM are at an increased risk of developing complications such as preeclampsia, cesarean delivery, and gestational hypertension. Furthermore, GDM is associated with adverse outcomes for the fetus, including macrosomia (excessive birth weight), neonatal hypoglycemia, and an increased likelihood of developing obesity and type 2 diabetes later in life.

The increasing prevalence of GDM is closely linked to the global rise in obesity and sedentary lifestyles. The condition has significant economic implications due to increased healthcare costs associated with managing maternal and neonatal complications. Therefore, addressing the prevention, early diagnosis, and effective management of GDM is crucial for both individual and public health.

Despite its prevalence and potential consequences, GDM remains a complex and challenging condition to manage. The understanding of its underlying mechanisms, risk factors, and optimal management strategies is continuously evolving. Advances in research and clinical practice have improved our ability to identify and manage GDM, but further efforts are required to optimize outcomes for women and their offspring.

This review aims to provide a comprehensive overview of GDM by examining its epidemiology, risk factors, pathophysiology, diagnostic criteria, complications, management strategies, and prevention approaches. By consolidating the current knowledge and highlighting recent advancements in the field, this review aims to contribute to the understanding and management of GDM, ultimately improving maternal and fetal health outcomes.

## Epidemiology and Risk Factors

Gestational Diabetes Mellitus (GDM) exhibits significant variation in prevalence among different populations and geographic regions worldwide. The condition affects approximately 7% of pregnancies globally, but this figure can vary substantially based on various factors, including ethnic background, socioeconomic status, and regional healthcare practices.

Certain ethnic backgrounds have been consistently associated with a higher risk of developing GDM. For instance, women of South Asian, Hispanic, African, and Native American descent have been shown to have an increased susceptibility to GDM compared to women of European ancestry. This ethnic disparity suggests a complex interplay of genetic, environmental, and lifestyle factors that contribute to GDM risk.

Maternal age is an important risk factor for GDM, with advanced maternal age (over 35 years) being associated with an increased likelihood of developing the condition. The age-related risk is believed to be linked to the natural decline in insulin sensitivity that occurs with aging, as well as an increased prevalence of obesity among older women.

Obesity is a well-established risk factor for GDM. Women with a pre-pregnancy body mass index (BMI) in the overweight or obese range are more likely to develop GDM compared to those with a healthy BMI. The excess adipose tissue in obesity promotes insulin resistance, impairing glucose regulation and increasing the risk of GDM.

A family history of diabetes is another important risk factor for GDM. Women with a parent or sibling diagnosed with diabetes have an elevated risk of developing GDM. Genetic factors, shared environmental influences, and lifestyle habits within families may contribute to this increased susceptibility.

Other risk factors for GDM include a previous history of GDM in a prior pregnancy, polycystic ovary syndrome (PCOS), and certain pregnancy-related conditions such as a history of macrosomia or unexplained stillbirth. Additionally, women with higher parity (number of previous pregnancies) may have an increased risk of GDM, although the underlying mechanisms for this association are not yet fully understood.

Understanding the epidemiology and risk factors of GDM is essential for identifying high-risk individuals and implementing preventive measures. Early identification and targeted interventions for women with known risk factors can help mitigate the development and adverse outcomes associated with GDM.

**Pathophysiology**

The pathophysiology of Gestational Diabetes Mellitus (GDM) involves a complex interplay of hormonal, metabolic, and inflammatory factors that collectively contribute to impaired glucose regulation during pregnancy. Understanding these underlying mechanisms is crucial for effective management and prevention of GDM.

Insulin resistance plays a central role in the development of GDM. Pregnancy induces physiological changes that lead to decreased insulin sensitivity in peripheral tissues, particularly in adipose tissue and skeletal muscle. The placenta produces various hormones, such as human placental lactogen (hPL), progesterone, and cortisol, which contribute to insulin resistance. These hormones interfere with insulin signaling pathways, impair glucose uptake by tissues, and promote lipolysis, resulting in increased circulating levels of free fatty acids.

β-cell dysfunction is another important aspect of GDM pathophysiology. While the insulin-secreting capacity of pancreatic β-cells usually increases to compensate for insulin resistance during pregnancy, in some women, β-cell function fails to adequately compensate, leading to insufficient insulin production. This inadequate response contributes to the persistent hyperglycemia observed in GDM.

Adipokines, which are adipose tissue-derived hormones, play a significant role in GDM pathophysiology. Increased levels of adipokines, such as adiponectin and resistin, have been observed in GDM. Adiponectin has insulin-sensitizing effects and is typically reduced in conditions of insulin resistance. Resistin, on the other hand, is pro-inflammatory and promotes insulin resistance. The dysregulation of adipokines contributes to the disturbed glucose metabolism seen in GDM.

Placental hormones, including hPL, insulin-like growth factor-1 (IGF-1), and leptin, also play a role in GDM development. These hormones modulate glucose and lipid metabolism, as well as insulin sensitivity, influencing fetal growth and nutrient availability. Imbalances in the production and action of these hormones can disrupt normal glucose regulation, contributing to GDM pathogenesis.

Inflammation has emerged as a potential contributor to GDM development. During pregnancy, there is a low-grade systemic inflammation characterized by increased levels of pro-inflammatory cytokines. This inflammatory state may impair insulin signaling and promote insulin resistance, further exacerbating glucose intolerance in GDM.

The precise mechanisms underlying the development of GDM remain an area of ongoing research. The complex interplay between genetic predisposition, hormonal changes, and metabolic factors during pregnancy contributes to the multifactorial nature of GDM pathophysiology. Further investigation is needed to unravel the intricate mechanisms involved and identify potential therapeutic targets for GDM prevention and management.

## Diagnostic Criteria

Early and accurate diagnosis of Gestational Diabetes Mellitus (GDM) is crucial for optimizing maternal and fetal outcomes. Various diagnostic criteria have been proposed to identify women with GDM, with the aim of detecting and managing the condition effectively.

The oral glucose tolerance test (OGTT) is the most widely accepted diagnostic method for GDM. Typically, a 2-step approach is employed. Initially, a non-fasting 50-gram glucose challenge test (GCT) is performed between 24 and 28 weeks of gestation. Blood glucose levels are measured one hour after consuming a glucose solution. If the result exceeds a specific threshold (typically 130-140 mg/dL), it is followed by a diagnostic OGTT.

The diagnostic OGTT involves fasting overnight followed by the administration of a 75-gram glucose load. Blood glucose levels are measured at fasting and at one, two, and three hours after glucose ingestion. The diagnostic thresholds for

GDM diagnosis based on the OGTT vary across different guidelines. Commonly used thresholds include fasting glucose ≥92-95 mg/dL, one-hour glucose ≥180-190 mg/dL, two-hour glucose ≥153-200 mg/dL, and three-hour glucose ≥140-145 mg/dL.

There has been ongoing controversy surrounding the diagnostic thresholds for GDM. Some argue for lower thresholds to capture milder forms of glucose intolerance and improve outcomes. Others argue for higher thresholds to avoid overdiagnosis and unnecessary interventions. As a result, different professional organizations and healthcare systems have adopted varying diagnostic criteria, leading to inconsistencies in the diagnosis and management of GDM.

In recent years, alternative screening approaches have been explored to simplify GDM diagnosis. One such approach is the use of fasting plasma glucose or random plasma glucose levels as a screening test, eliminating the need for the initial GCT. However, these approaches have not been universally adopted, and the OGTT remains the gold standard for GDM diagnosis in most settings.

The importance of universal screening for GDM is widely recognized. Universal screening aims to identify all women with GDM, including those who are asymptomatic or do not possess obvious risk factors. This approach ensures early detection and appropriate management of GDM, thereby reducing the risk of maternal and fetal complications. However, the feasibility and cost-effectiveness of universal screening have been subjects of debate, particularly in resource-limited settings.

In conclusion, the diagnostic criteria for GDM primarily involve the oral glucose tolerance test (OGTT) following a glucose challenge test (GCT). The specific thresholds for diagnosing GDM vary across different guidelines, leading to controversy and inconsistencies in diagnostic approaches. Alternative screening approaches have been explored, but the OGTT remains the gold standard. Universal screening is considered crucial for early detection and optimal management of GDM, although the feasibility and cost-effectiveness of this approach are still debated.

## Maternal and Fetal Complications

Gestational Diabetes Mellitus (GDM) poses significant risks to both the mother and the fetus. Proper management of GDM is crucial to mitigate these complications and improve outcomes for both.

## Maternal Complications

**Preeclampsia:** Women with GDM have an increased risk of developing preeclampsia, a condition characterized by high blood pressure and organ damage. Preeclampsia can lead to complications such as preterm birth, placental abruption, and maternal organ dysfunction.

**Cesarean Delivery:** GDM is associated with a higher likelihood of cesarean delivery. This may be due to factors such as macrosomia, fetal distress, or failed induction of labor.

**Gestational Hypertension:** GDM increases the risk of developing gestational hypertension, a condition characterized by high blood pressure during pregnancy. This can lead to complications for both the mother and the baby if left uncontrolled.

**Increased Risk of Type 2 Diabetes:** Women with a history of GDM are at an increased risk of developing type 2 diabetes later in life. Approximately 50% of women with GDM will develop type 2 diabetes within 5-10 years after pregnancy. Regular follow-up and lifestyle modifications are essential to reduce this long-term risk.

**Fetal and Neonatal Complications:**

**Macrosomia:** Babies born to mothers with uncontrolled GDM are at risk of macrosomia, which refers to excessive birth weight. This can lead to birth injuries, such as shoulder dystocia, and an increased risk of cesarean delivery.

**Neonatal Hypoglycemia:** Infants of mothers with GDM may experience low blood sugar levels (hypoglycemia) shortly after birth. This is because the baby's pancreas may have adapted to the higher blood glucose levels in utero and continues to produce high insulin levels after delivery. Prompt monitoring and management of blood glucose levels in the newborn are crucial to prevent complications.

**Respiratory Distress Syndrome:** Babies born to mothers with GDM are at an increased risk of respiratory distress syndrome, a condition characterized by breathing difficulties due to immature lungs. This can necessitate specialized medical care and support for the newborn.

**Increased Risk of Obesity and Type 2 Diabetes:** Children born to mothers with GDM have a higher risk of developing obesity and type 2 diabetes later in life. It emphasizes the importance of lifestyle modifications, breastfeeding, and regular monitoring of the child's health.

It is essential to note that appropriate management of GDM through lifestyle modifications, blood sugar monitoring, and, in some cases, medication can significantly reduce the risks of these complications. Regular prenatal care, close monitoring, and collaboration between healthcare providers are crucial to optimizing outcomes for both the mother and the baby.

## Management Strategies

The management of Gestational Diabetes Mellitus (GDM) focuses on achieving and maintaining optimal blood glucose control to reduce the risk of complications for both the mother and the fetus. It requires a multidisciplinary approach involving healthcare professionals, including obstetricians, endocrinologists, dietitians, and diabetes educators.

Lifestyle Interventions: Lifestyle modifications form the cornerstone of GDM management and often serve as the first-line treatment approach. These interventions include:

Medical Nutrition Therapy: Individualized meal plans tailored to the woman's nutritional needs are developed in collaboration with a registered dietitian. The goals of medical nutrition therapy are to achieve appropriate weight gain, promote healthy blood glucose levels, and ensure adequate fetal nutrition. It typically involves consuming a well-balanced diet with controlled carbohydrate intake, spread across multiple meals and snacks throughout the day.

Regular Physical Activity: Engaging in regular physical activity, as recommended by healthcare providers, can help improve insulin sensitivity and blood glucose control. Women with GDM are generally encouraged to engage in moderate-intensity aerobic exercise, such as walking or swimming, for at least 150 minutes per week, unless contraindicated.

Blood Glucose Monitoring: Regular self-monitoring of blood glucose levels is a crucial component of GDM management. It involves using a glucometer to measure blood sugar levels before and after meals. Healthcare providers guide women on the target blood glucose ranges to maintain, aiming for fasting levels $\leq 95$ mg/dL and either one-hour postprandial levels ≤140 mg/dL or two-hour postprandial levels ≤120 mg/dL. Monitoring helps assess the effectiveness of lifestyle modifications and enables adjustments in treatment plans if necessary.

Pharmacological Interventions: a. Oral Hypoglycemic Agents: If lifestyle modifications alone do not achieve target blood glucose levels, oral hypoglycemic agents, such as metformin or glyburide, may be prescribed. These medications help lower blood sugar levels and are considered safe for use during pregnancy, although they require careful monitoring and supervision by healthcare providers.

b. Insulin Therapy: Insulin remains the most effective and commonly used treatment option for GDM if blood glucose targets cannot be achieved with lifestyle modifications and oral hypoglycemic agents or in cases where oral medications are contraindicated. Insulin therapy may involve multiple daily injections or the use of insulin pumps to maintain optimal blood glucose control.

Regular follow-up visits with healthcare providers are essential throughout the pregnancy to monitor blood glucose levels, assess fetal growth, and make any necessary adjustments to the treatment plan. Delivery plans are individualized based on maternal and fetal well-being, and coordination with the obstetric team is crucial to ensure a safe and successful delivery.

Education and support from healthcare professionals, including diabetes self-management education, play a vital role in empowering women with GDM to manage their condition effectively. Ongoing support and follow-up after delivery are also crucial to screen for persistent glucose intolerance and provide counseling on lifestyle modifications to reduce the long-term risk of type 2 diabetes.

**Prevention and Screening**

Efforts to prevent GDM and identify high-risk individuals are crucial in reducing its burden. This section explores various preventive measures, including lifestyle interventions, pharmacological approaches, and early identification of women at risk. The potential benefits of preconception counseling and interventions are also discussed.

## Recent Advances and Future Directions

This section highlights recent advancements in the understanding and management of GDM. Topics covered include the use of continuous glucose monitoring, personalized medicine approaches, the role of gut microbiota, and the potential for targeted therapies. It also identifies areas that require further research to improve the prevention, diagnosis, and treatment of GDM.

**Conclusion**

Gestational Diabetes Mellitus is a significant health concern affecting a substantial number of pregnant women worldwide. This narrative review provides a comprehensive overview of GDM, encompassing its epidemiology, risk factors, pathophysiology, diagnostic criteria, complications, management, and prevention strategies. By improving our understanding of GDM and implementing effective management strategies, we can enhance the health outcomes for both the mother and the offspring and reduce the long-term risk of type 2 diabetes.

Disclaimer: This review is based on the available literature up until September 2021. It is essential to consult current guidelines and medical literature for the most up-to-date information on the subject.

**References**

1. American Diabetes Association. (2021). Standards of Medical Care in Diabetes—2021. Diabetes Care, 44(Supplement 1), S1–S232.

2. Buckley, B. S., Harreiter, J., Damm, P., Corcoy, R., Chico, A., Simmons, D., Vellinga, A., Dunne, F., & Group, G. D. S. (2012). Gestational diabetes mellitus in Europe: prevalence, current screening practice and barriers to screening. A review. Diabetic Medicine, 29(7), 844–854.

3. Metzger, B. E., & Lowe, L. P. (2008). Hyperglycemia and adverse pregnancy outcomes. New England Journal of Medicine, 358(19), 1991–2002.

4. Lain, K. Y., & Catalano, P. M. (2007). Metabolic changes in pregnancy. Clinical Obstetrics and Gynecology, 50(4), 938–948.

5. Sacks, D. A., Hadden, D. R., Maresh, M., Deerochanawong, C., Dyer, A. R.,

Metzger, B. E., Lowe, L. P., &
Coustan, D. R. (2012). Frequency of
gestational diabetes mellitus at
collaborating centers based on
IADPSG consensus panel–
recommended criteria: The
Hyperglycemia and Adverse
Pregnancy Outcome (HAPO) study.
Diabetes Care, 35(3), 526–528.

6. American College of Obstetricians and
Gynecologists. (2018). ACOG practice
bulletin no. 190: Gestational diabetes
mellitus. Obstetrics and Gynecology,
131(2), e49–e64.

7. Reece, E. A., Leguizamón, G., &
Wiznitzer, A. (2009). Gestational
diabetes: the need for a common

ground. Lancet, 373(9677), 1789–1797.

8. Farrar, D., Simmonds, M., Bryant, M., Sheldon, T. A., Tuffnell, D., Golder, S., Dunne, F., & Lawlor, D. A. (2016). Hyperglycaemia and risk of adverse perinatal outcomes: systematic review and meta-analysis. BMJ, 354, i4694.

9. American Diabetes Association. (2021). 14. Management of Diabetes in Pregnancy: Standards of Medical Care in Diabetes—2021. Diabetes Care, 44(Supplement 1), S200–S210.

10.     Cho, N. H., Shaw, J. E., Karuranga, S., Huang, Y., da Rocha Fernandes, J. D., Ohlrogge, A. W., Malanda, B., & IDF Diabetes Atlas Committee. (2018). IDF Diabetes

Atlas: Global estimates of diabetes prevalence for 2017 and projections for 2045. Diabetes Research and Clinical Practice, 138, 271–281.

11.     Metzger, B. E., Gabbe, S. G., Persson, B., Buchanan, T. A., Catalano, P. M., Damm, P., ... & Hod, M. (2010). International association of diabetes and pregnancy study groups recommendations on the diagnosis and classification of hyperglycemia in pregnancy. Diabetes Care, 33(3), 676-682.

12.     HAPO Study Cooperative Research Group. (2008). Hyperglycemia and Adverse Pregnancy Outcome (HAPO) Study: Associations with neonatal

anthropometrics. Diabetes, 58(2), 453-459.

13.     Landon, M. B., Spong, C. Y., Thom, E., Carpenter, M. W., Ramin, S. M., Casey, B., ... & Sciscione, A. (2009). A multicenter, randomized trial of treatment for mild gestational diabetes. New England Journal of Medicine, 361(14), 1339-1348.

14.     American Diabetes Association. (2020). 14. Management of Diabetes in Pregnancy: Standards of Medical Care in Diabetes—2020. Diabetes Care, 43(Supplement 1), S183-S192.

15.     Hod, M., Kapur, A., Sacks, D. A., Hadar, E., Agarwal, M., Di Renzo, G. C., ... & McIntyre, H. D. (2020). The International Federation of

Gynecology and Obstetrics (FIGO) initiative on gestational diabetes mellitus: A pragmatic guide for diagnosis, management, and care. International Journal of Gynecology & Obstetrics, 149(Supplement 3), 2-21.

16.	American College of Obstetricians and Gynecologists. (2021). ACOG Practice Bulletin No. 225: Gestational Diabetes Mellitus. Obstetrics & Gynecology, 137(2), e49-e64.

17.	Zhang, C., Rawal, S., & Chong, Y. S. (2018). Risk factors for gestational diabetes: is prevention possible? Diabetologia, 61(5), 962-969.

18.	Moses, R. G., Wong, V. C., Lambert, K., Morris, G. J., San Gil, F., & Lowe, J. (2020). The prevalence of hyperglycaemia in pregnancy in Australia: a national 3-year cross-sectional study. The Medical Journal of Australia, 213(2), 71-77.

19.	Tieu, J., Shepherd, E., Middleton, P., Crowther, C. A., & Group, A. T. (2017). Dietary advice interventions in pregnancy for preventing gestational diabetes mellitus. Cochrane Database of Systematic Reviews, (1), CD006674.

20.	Collier, A., Abraham, E. C., Armstrong, J., & Dornhorst, A. (2020). Guidelines for the prevention and management of diabetes in pregnancy:

time to improve our approach?
Diabetic Medicine, 37(9), 1501-1509

21.     McIntyre, H. D., Catalano, P., Zhang, C., Desoye, G., Mathiesen, E. R., Damm, P., ... & Hod, M. (2019). Gestational diabetes mellitus. Nature Reviews Disease Primers, 5(1), 1-22.

22.     Lowe, W. L., & Scholtens, D. M. (2020). Hyperglycemia in pregnancy and future risk of diabetes: How do we balance the evidence? Diabetes Care, 43(11), 2649-2652.

23.     Kapur, A., & Hadden, D. R. (2017). Gestational diabetes mellitus: Indian perspective. Journal of the Indian Medical Association, 115(2), 111-114.

24.     Ferrara, A. (2007). Increasing prevalence of gestational diabetes mellitus: a public health perspective. Diabetes Care, 30(Supplement 2), S141-S146.

25.     Cho, N. H., Shaw, J. E., Karuranga, S., Huang, Y., da Rocha Fernandes, J. D., Ohlrogge, A. W., ... & Malanda, B. (2018). IDF Diabetes Atlas: Global estimates of diabetes prevalence for 2017 and projections for 2045. Diabetes Research and Clinical Practice, 138, 271-281.

26.     Zhu, Y., Zhang, C. (2020). Prevalence of gestational diabetes and risk of progression to type 2 diabetes: a global perspective. Current Diabetes Reports, 20(1), 1-10.

27.     Koivusalo, S. B., Rönö, K., Klemetti, M. M., Roine, R. P., Lindström, J., Erkkola, M., ... & Pöyhönen-Alho, M. (2016). Gestational diabetes mellitus can be prevented by lifestyle intervention: The Finnish Gestational Diabetes Prevention Study (RADIEL): a randomized controlled trial. Diabetes Care, 39(1), 24-30.